AROMATHERAPY AND ESSENTIAL OILS

THE ULTIMATE GUIDE TO ESSENTIAL OILS FOR HEALING AND ESSENTIAL OILS RECIPES

ADAHI FLORES

CONTENTS

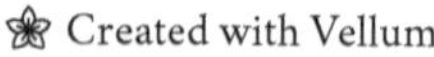 Created with Vellum

INTRODUCTION

This book contains proven steps and strategies for choosing the correct essential oil based on its properties and desire results. It also has a sample recipe mix for essential oils that will surely make your everyday fragrant, relaxing, and germ-free.

As you will see in this book, Aromatherapy, the art, and science of using essential oils for a purpose that will give a better quality of life, has been around since ancient times in several parts of the globe but is still a favorite subject among scientific studies and research. It's not just that almost magical scents of these oils that perked our senses and insistence for truth and knowledge, which makes the subject of tempting aromatherapy medical-wise. But the various properties that are potent enough to provide us with confidence to seek the natural way of preventing or treating disease—healing our scarred physical, mental, and emotional systems, and strengthening our health and longevity in general.

You must have your reasons for holding this book, and whatever it is, I hope that I will be of help. This book intends to cater to various people – a budding esthetician, hobbyist, student, or just a curious book finder. So, the words are written in a format that is understandable from a layman's perspective. But, on the other hand, it lacks the technicality of manuals and handbooks that explore essential oils' chemical formulations, structures, and biochemical effects. Hence, if you are a beginner who wants to get involved in the wonderful world of aromatics and essential oils, then I can assure you that you have come to the right place to start.

HISTORY OF AROMATHERAPY

What You Need to Know about Essential Oils' Beginnings

The exact beginning of Aromatherapy is impossible to determine. Historians can only logically point to the possibility that Aromatherapy is an accident in its discovery just after the discovery of fire. On the other hand, earth and man probably witnessed the birth of Aromatherapy when the latter became more adept in making fire out of dry wood, leaves, and any of Mother Nature's flammable materials. In one of his amateurish pyrotechnics, he might have used cedar or cypress as firewood or burned tree saps or resin, from which a unique, fragrant scent arose. However, it is very similar to a type of Aromatherapy we now referred to as incense.

Prehistorically. A stroke of luck only discovered incense – it doesn't serve any purpose. However, the Neolithic Era and the Age of Ancient Civilizations have seen the great importance of scent in everyday life and culture and used it for various purposes, including religious ceremonies, relaxation, and healing.

From 7000 – 4000 BC, two other vital pieces of knowledge in Aromatherapy still exist today are mixing plant parts with heated animal fats to produce a scented fat containing the plant's unique aromatics, protective elements, etc. healing and energizing properties. This practice is the origin of modern massage oil and lotion. Another is the creation of aromatic water from plant oils and alcohol mixed in water. Such substance for consumption as a medicinal tonic during ancient times, but its form, properties, and concoction methods are akin to those of present-day perfumes.

The history of Aromatherapy comes from unearthed Egyptian stone tablets. For example, one mural adorning Queen Hatshepsut's temple walls portrays sacks of frankincense traded from Pwenet or the historical Land of Punt. Even Imhotep, an Egyptian, a doctor, and priest credited as the grandfather of Aromatherapy, used these methods. Archaeologists also reported that the tomb of Tutankhamen filled the air with scents of spikenard and myrrh when opened.

These pieces of evidence show that the Egyptians were far more advanced and established with the use of essential oils. Aromatherapy was an indispensable part of their lives. It was not limited to royalties and the members of high society – even commoners could use it. Frankincense such as myrrh, jasmine, cassia oils, and cedarwood for religious ceremonies. Or rituals and mummification, and as an alternative for healing, and toiletries. Fragrant oils were also added to the bath to improve the beauty, refresh the mind, and lift the moods, or applied to the body as perfume and protection against the harsh sun and climate.

. . .

Frankincense fragrances. Such as myrrh and other oils from saffron, spikenard, lilies, and cinnamon herbs. They lie depicted in the Old Testament, particularly in Isaiah and Solomon's song. The Hebrews brought with them the practice of using plant and animal oils and essences from the Egyptians when they returned to Israel after the Exodus. The Greeks obtained knowledge from the Egyptians, and both civilizations considered the fragrant plant essences as gods' gifts to men. Romans, in turn, learned it from the Greeks. Perfumes were like a fashion trend in the Roman Empire. Simultaneously, China learned of the art through trade with other civilizations.

Ancients used Aromatherapy for therapeutic purposes known as Ayurveda, traditionally practiced in India for at least 3,000 years. Ancient Hindu texts suggested that sandalwood, myrrh, ginger, rose, and coriander in use as fragrances during rituals. India is the birthplace of Buddhism and Hinduism. Both religions knew incense to honor gods and drive away demons and evil spirits.

Aromatherapy reached the lands of Europe following the return of Crusaders who traveled to the Holy Land. It became a craft and livelihood throughout the Middle Ages, particularly in Grasse, France, a city tagged as the world's perfume capital. Therefore, it's no surprise that the person who prominently worked to reintroduce and finally stabilize the health and medical importance of Aromatherapy in the Modern era is a French "essential oil" connoisseur.

Rene Maurice Gattefosse, a cosmetologist and chemist, studied essential oils' antibiotic and disinfecting properties for more than

50 years. He began testing his theories in 1936 after accidentally burning his arm and personally witnessing the power of lavender oil to lessen the pain of his burns and cure them quickly. As a result, he was the one who first used the term "aromatherapy," which is Aromatherapy in French.

Other experts have followed Gattefosse's theories and work hitherto. Gattefosse's colleague Godissart introduced Aromatherapy in the US as a treatment of severe diseases. In the 1950s, French biochemist Marguerite Maury suggested that the body best absorbed essential oils through massage. Together with Micheline Arcier, she started several European clinics that offered personally concocted blends to treat each patient's specific illness.

After taking a down-time due to the rise to fame of synthetic drugs in the field of medicine, Aromatherapy re-entered the mainstream as a natural way of curing disease. As of present, it is one of the most sought-after alternatives to disease treatment and an indispensable element in areas of beauty, cosmetics, and stress relief.

HOW AROMATHERAPY AND ESSENTIAL OILS WORK THEIR MAGIC

Essential oils possess properties that give potent reactions to the body in physical, mental, and even spiritual aspects. They are powerful energy and immune system stimulants and relaxants with antiseptic, analgesic, and antidepressant properties. Due to these properties, essential oils are now an indispensable item in healing practices, particularly in treating physical wounds, pains, skin infections, and even psychological illnesses such as depression and insomnia. Essential oils can reestablish the balance in hormones and body energies (chakras) at a cellular level. They can also significantly relieve stress and personal issues like low self-esteem, grief, and low moods.

The common idea in modern medicine is 1 compound, say aspirin, equals one batch of properties that will serve the compound's healing purpose. Essential oil, on the other hand, is a mixture of different combinations with unique sets of properties. Yet despite this diversity of compounds in a single substance, essential oil and its various therapeutic effects can work synergistically and supply what the body needs from it. But how can these oils work their magic, technically speaking?

. . .

Essential oils can naturally increase oxygen amounts in the air in a closed and narrow space. In a layman's chemistry version, essential oils boost the ozone and negative ions in a given atmosphere, inhibiting bacterial growth and the foul odors from microbial build-ups. They can also get easily attracted to chemical bonds of toxic chemicals present in the air, destroying them and making them safe and breathable. Essential oils remove poisonous substances from the body in the same way, i.e., organically binding with toxins and forming new substances. The body can easily flush the substances out of the body.

Essential oils can successfully get inside us through our olfactory, digestive and integumentary (skin) systems. Probably the oldest and most well-known medium through which essential oils combine to give the desired effects to the body is the olfactory system. Particularly the nose since, as already mentioned, it's highly probable (and logical) that Aromatherapy was first discovered in the form of incense – a fragrant, relaxing scent coming from a burning botanical source. In the eventual rise of civilizations and the formation of cities, cultures, and technologies, essential oils became revered in areas of health and beauty, utilized not only as burned incenses but also as ingestible solutions and topical salves.

Integumentary System

The human skin is the biggest organ that acts as the body's protection against damaging agents from the outside. It contains millions of openings where hair protrudes – a system that adds up to its natural permeability. Like hormone replacement creams and nicotine patches, these oils blend into the skin. The absorption and effects at the cellular level can be significantly hastened, usually within 20 minutes, thru massaging or rubbing. The heat and controlled movements in the area increase blood and oxygen circulation, enhancing the absorption of essential oils.

According to some studies, the absorption rate is faster in body areas where the sweat glands and hair follicles concentrate, specifically in the genitalia, palms, soles of the feet, head, and armpits.

Olfactory System

The olfactory system is the group of organs or cells that work together to carry out the functions and processes contributing to or related to the sense and perception of scent. This system's most utilized and probably official member is the nose and its parts, though the mouth can transport these scents.

When we inhale through the nose or mouth, airborne molecules possessing odors travel through the opening and interact with olfactory organs that simultaneously transport signals to the brain. The brain has several receptor sites, but the location of interest is the limbic system, also known as the "emotional brain." The limbic system works with the other brain parts that regulate heart rate, breathing, hormone balance, and blood pressure.

This connection is the main reason why electrochemical messages received by the limbic system can significantly trigger emotions and memories. On the outside, we usually associate smells with specific events in our lives. The trigger and release of sedating or stimulating neurochemicals via the use of essential oils take advantage of this process, providing such profound influence on our physiological and psychological systems and functions.

The odor molecules don't just stop in the brain but travel to the lungs and parts of the respiratory system. Therefore, it is safe to say that the effects of essential oils can reach other parts of the body through several pathways. For example, inhaling peppermint is widely practiced reducing dizziness and fatigue, and eucalyptus is great for treating coughs and sore throat.

Digestive System

Another main pathway through which essential oils enter the body is via ingestion or swallowing. Drinking concocted essential oils was practiced since the glorious days of the Egyptian, Greek, and Roman civilizations.

However, the public is discouraged by experts from ingesting essential oils due to the limitations of studies and experiments in knowledge regarding its safety if swallowed directly in concentrated amounts. Some studies declare that some essential oils can damage the digestive system, particularly if denatured by gastric processes. Others claim that these plant oils can significantly toxically eat significant organs like the liver and kidneys. In addition, doctors discourage ingestion of essential oils for patients who regularly intake meds for their specific illnesses because the compounds in these oils can potentially weaken or damage such drugs' effectiveness or combine with the chemicals in drugs to produce a fatal product. As of present, there are few groups of people who believe in the efficacy of essential oil application through ingestion, albeit practiced only under the strict guidance of expert physicians or pharmacists.

3

BASIC ESSENTIAL OIL KIT

The essential oil contains at least 100 different components, including terpenes, ketones, phenols, alcohols, aldehydes, and esters. These substances, despite their sweet-smelling nature, are highly complex and potent. As a result, they have a wide range of uses and importance, from food and gardening to treating common ailments and serious diseases. Types of essential oils are almost as many as the number of plant species on this planet. And while each has unique beneficial properties, only 10 of them are widely used and considered a must-have in everyone's home Eucalyptus, peppermint, geranium, rosemary, tea tree, chamomile, thyme, lavender, clove, and lemon. If you're a novice in the world of Aromatherapy, acquiring these essential oils will be a great way to start.

Eucalyptus

Highly potent and versatile, eucalyptus has been extracted since the 1700s in Australia, specifically in the Blue Mountains in New South Wales, where the mountains and the whole landscape lie covered by a blue haze exuded by the plant's gum resins. Eucalyptus gets its value for its effectiveness in treating colic, cough, cold, and joint, respiratory illnesses.

Research, however, has found that eucalyptus packs more prowess, including antiviral, anti-inflammatory, analgesic, antiseptic, deodorizing, and diuretic properties. Effective in fighting off flu and reducing muscular pains, eucalyptus also has properties substantially potent in treating diabetes, candida, cystitis, and skin problems. In addition, it is a powerful insect repellent and skin protector against weather extremes. Although widely used and applied, a pregnant woman should not use eucalyptus.

Peppermint

Peppermint is a common ingredient in toothpaste, mouthwash, and breath-freshening gums nowadays. It is essential to know that peppermint has been employed since the ancient period because of its antiseptic properties, specifically by the Chinese, Egyptian, and Native Americans? Peppermint is also an effective anti-inflammatory used to cure toothaches and gum bleeding.

Peppermint is a widely used essential oil not only because of its cool and clean scent that makes it a favorite breath freshener and mouth cleaner. More than that, it has antispasmodic properties that make it effective in dealing with rheumatoid arthritis, muscle aches, tendonitis, and abdominal pains. Peppermint is also helpful and potent in conditions like nausea, dysmenorrhea, hemorrhoids, heatstroke, flatulence, headaches, hay fever, respiratory illnesses such as bronchitis, sinusitis, colds and flu, also digestive problems such as constipation, and indigestion, and skin conditions such as rashes, sunburns, fungal infections, itching, and scabies.

Although peppermint is naturally safe and non-toxic, it can irritate or burn the skin in concentrated amounts. Hence, it must not be applied directly to the skin in pure, somewhat diluted initially with another oil, preferably nut or seed oil.

Geranium

Geranium extracted from the Geranium Robert plant, also known as the "lemon plant," of the Pelargonium species. Particularly a favorite in dealing with women's health conditions. From dysmenorrhea to menopausal problems to endometriosis. It has powerful sedating and pain-reducing effects.

Geranium is a widely used ingredient in skin products. Anecdotal evidence claim that geranium application can cure blisters overnight and provide radiant and glowing skin if used regularly. It has also been found effective in treating acne, burns, bruises, and spider veins.

Health conditions are either reduced or eliminated by the geranium essential oil. For example, geranium can treat sore throat, diabetes, high blood pressure, hormonal imbalances, ringworm, insomnia, hemorrhoids, and liver congestion.

Rosemary

. . .

Rosemary is not just an excellent spice to occupy a significant portion of your kitchen. Its essential oil works wonders in both mental and physical health. Aside from the positive results in treating muscular pains, sprains, arthritis, rheumatism, migraines, and respiratory illnesses, it also aids patients suffering from psychological conditions such as depression and dementia.

It also has stimulating properties, making it a good choice for an additive to a nice, relaxing bath after a long, tiring day. It will surely make your mornings energized and your whole day stress-less.

Rosemary is also a favorite in men's and women's beauty regimens, indispensable in hair and skincare. It is effective in curing acne, eczema, dandruff, dermatitis, fungal infections, cellulitis, varicose veins, and hair loss. People with high blood pressure and epilepsy, however, should stay away from it.

Tea Tree

Tea tree has been a subject of a lot of research then and now. It has a list of impressive properties, particularly its antiseptic prowess that is 100% more potent than carbolic acid in dealing with a wide range of harmful bacteria, viruses, and fungi, minus the toxicity. Because of this quality, the tea tree becomes indispensable in treating acne, fungal infections, sunburns, body odor, and candida.

Chamomile

. . .

There are several species of chamomile, but the most widely used and probably most potent is chamomile German. Another good variety is chamomile Roman. Although above par in terms of antiseptic and disinfecting qualities, chamomile is best known for its anti-inflammatory properties, effective in dealing with internal and external inflammations.

It is a desirable skin rejuvenating ingredient, even curing fungal infections like boils and ringworm and harsh skin conditions like sunburns, eczema, and psoriasis. Chamomile is also an indispensable item in childcare since it is a safe additive in baby baths and has good teething support. In addition, its calming effects make it a great aid in stabilizing patients in either nervous or depressive states.

Thyme

Thyme is always a partner of rosemary. Together, they form the herb de Provence that is a staple in the kitchens of Europe. The essential oil extracted from thyme is a potent insect and parasite repellent. In addition, thyme is a good antiseptic, antiviral, antibacterial, and diuretic component that can treat various diseases and health conditions. These include superficial wounds and skin abrasions, fungal infections, constipation, bronchitis, colds, flu, cough, dandruff, bladder infections, arthritis, and arteriosclerosis.

The action of thyme is so intense that it requires extreme care during handling and application. Pure, concentrated thyme must not be applied to the skin because it can cause severe irritation and extreme sensitization to sunlight. In addition, the user must monitor its use since overuse can lead to thyroid and lymphatic problems. Therefore, high dilution is necessary before application. Thyme is also not advised for children's use.

Lavender

Lavender is an all-time favorite of all essential oils. Its light, fragrant scent produces both energizing and calming effects on the moods. Therefore, a recommendation is that each home has this essential oil due to its potent antiseptic properties if no other oil is available. In addition, based on research and personal anecdotes, lavender can significantly detoxify and stimulate cell regeneration, which is particularly helpful in treating wounds and preventing scarring.

Lavender is also a powerful sedative that can stabilize moods and the state of mind after a shock.

Clove

Aside from being a space that's regularly incorporated in meals, clove has highly antiseptic, analgesic, and antibacterial essential oil that can be very helpful in the treatment and prevention of diseases and infections. Its painkilling properties work for toothaches, muscle pains, and digestive problems. Its antiseptic quality is so potent that clove is efficient in the sterilization of surgical instruments. In addition, it's an effective cure for common conditions like flu, sinusitis, and nausea.

Lemon

. . .

Lemon saved many sailors in history due to its rich vitamin C content that cured scurvy. In addition, lemon strengthens the immune system and fight common flu, colds, coughs, sore throat, and tonsillitis. Lemon is a favorite. Lemon is a die-hard dieter, a natural diuretic and metabolizing aid, can burn fat and dispersing cellulitis fast. Its fragrant smell works good on humans' noses but is repulsive to insects and parasites. Its potent antiseptic and antibacterial properties help fight mouth ulcers, intestinal parasites, bronchitis, boils, warts, and acne. Lemon oil, however, is not recommended for children's use.

4

THE ROLE OF AROMATHERAPY AND ESSENTIAL OILS TO MODERN LIFE AND HEALTH

If somebody asks you what Aromatherapy is, what is the first thing that would come to your mind? Considering that you've read about it. On lifestyle magazines. Or you've seen them in services offered in spas and massage clinics. You'll probably think or say that Aromatherapy is a relaxing procedure wherein fragrant. Calming oils are either massaged to the body or allowed to be breathed in for a few hours. It is correct, but there's more to Aromatherapy than its mood-enhancing and relaxing effects. Aromatherapy is more expansive and encompassing than you could expect it to be.

For instance, as historical records tell us, essential oils are also known for their medicinal uses. Since these oils are plant aromatics, they naturally possess anti-inflammatory, analgesic, and antiseptic properties. Even Hippocrates, the father of medicine, claimed that bathing in essential oils every day could promote overall health and prevent the acquirement of diseases. Modern society believes in Aromatherapy potentials as much as the generations of old, or probably a bit more, because numerous scientific studies continuously discover the ultimate power behind Aromatherapy and how it works. Aromatherapy has the potential to cure some of the most harmful diseases we have today. This chapter will discuss the indispensable role of Aromatherapy in the modern health and lifestyle scenario.

Beauty and Skin Health

Beauty, contrary to the famous saying, is not skin deep. We will not discuss the true meaning of this idiomatic expression here, i.e., true beauty is the kindness of the heart, but rather focus on the other applicable purpose of this expression about health. Beauty, in an evolutionary aspect, is a real sign of good genes and solid reproductive health. For instance, the male bird of paradise, a bird endemic in the natural rainforests of Papua New Guinea, displays its bright-colored feathers to attract a potential mate. Male hippos fight viciously for a female mate with their long, deadly teeth. The stronger and more vicious will win and get the prize. Eventually, the family line of every species continues again through the birth of offspring.

The standard of physical beauty varies from every species, but one thing is sure: strength and vitality, which mirror the best of health, are always synonymous with beauty. Good health reflects on the outside. For humans, beauty is characterized by whatever manifests on the outside, specifically on the skin, the human body's largest organ. Marks, bruises, or rashes that mar the skin's flawlessness are ugly and tell-tale signs of disease or infection.

So why are essential oils vital to acquiring and maintaining skin health and beauty? Essential oils are well, although their consistency is like that of water or alcohol, and they are not as greasy as common vegetable oils and animal fats. They're also somewhat lighter in both appearance and texture. If you're familiar with the natural facial serums, we have nowadays. Then you have an idea of what essential oils look and feel like. These properties of essential oils make them potent moisturizers that can prevent early signs of aging like wrinkles, crow's feet, and frequent dryness. For example, the Egyptian queen renowned for her beauty and flawless complexion, Cleopatra, is reputedly bathed in milk with rose petals and jasmine oil every day. Therefore, is quite a feat for the queen, considering that Egypt has a sweltering climate and is mostly desert sand.

Essential oils do not just act on the outer layer of skin. Still, they are absorbed into the dermis, as researchers have found that crucial oil contents are present in breath, sweat, urine, and other excretory products. In addition, massage makes the absorption of essential oils by the skin more accessible and faster.

Based on findings, essential oils can stimulate skin renewal and rejuvenation faster, wherein old skin is eliminated, and new skin grows more quickly than average. Massaging with essential oils also promotes good blood circulation, which removes toxins accumulated in the lymphatic glands. Both qualities result in younger, firmer, and suppler skin.

Essential oils, as mentioned, possess natural antibiotic and anti-inflammatory properties, which can neutralize the negative actions of harmful microbes on the skin and calm damaged skin. Greeks and Romans used to ingest blends of essential oils as a health drink that cures skin illnesses. Nowadays, even anti-aging creams and serums contain essential oils, too.

· · ·

ANTI-AGING

Choose from the following essential oils:

Rose
Lavender
Patchouli
Geranium
Chamomile
Lemon
Oregano
Orange
Rosemary
Lime
Carrot
Thyme
Neroli
Fennel
Clary-sage
Violet Leaf

As Facial Cleanser: Mix 60mL spring or distilled water. 60mL apple cider vinegar (organic) and six drops of any essential oil of your choice.

If you want your cleanser to be oil-based, add in 90mL of either almond or avocado oil or a mixture of 45mL avocado oil and 45mL almond oil.

Place inside a sterilized glass jar or vessel and store in a cool, dry place.

. . .

As Face and Body Rub: Dilute 30 drops of the chosen essential oil into two tablespoons of nut oil (almond, hazelnut, or apricot kernel). Rub the final product lightly and thinly on the face and neck at night, just after washing and drying the face.

You can also mix different essential oils before diluting them in the nut oil; make sure that everything will sum up to 30 drops of essential oil. For example, mix one drop of carrot, three drops of chamomile, five drops of lavender and fennel, and eight drops of geranium and neroli before diluting the resulting mixture to 2 tablespoons of nut oil.

As for Bath Solution: Add 6 – 10 drops of the selected essential oil into the bath.

Robust Immune System and Disease Treatment

Aromatherapy, according to research, is an effective immune system booster. For example, essential oils absorbed by the body through either an olfactory introduction or topical application can cure people suffering from common flu and colds. In addition, the healing properties of many essential oils significantly decrease the workload of our immune system. One research even revealed that essential oils stimulate the production and release of white corpuscles, indispensable in the body's defense against diseases.

The combined potential of essential oils and lymphatic massage effectively removes toxins from the body. Lymph nodes are anatomically and physiologically crucial to maintain an optimum immune system. Thanks to the capability of the said organs to filter out toxins present in the blood. Coincidentally, these lymphatic nodes are present in the body where sweat glands and hair concentrate (armpits, genitals, soles, and palms), implying that lymphatic massage involves deep strokes in the muscles that expedite the body's absorption of essential oils. Therefore, lemon and grapefruit essential oils are indispensable for this blood cleansing procedure. Moreover, the said crucial oils are abundant in Vitamin C, necessary for building a robust immune system.

The health benefits of essential oils originate from their antiseptic, analgesic, anti-inflammatory, diuretic, antibacterial, antifungal, antiviral, disinfecting, and detoxifying properties. These properties largely contribute to preventing and treating diseases like ordinary flu, colds, and skin infections. However, more and more academic research shows strong proof of essential oils' significance in treating the severe illnesses of this generation, particularly depression, candidiasis, and even cancers.

For Flu, Colds, and Other Viral Illnesses: Essential oils are nonselective agents, meaning they can disrupt molecular targets regardless of any changes in a specific protein. That's why the ability of viruses to develop susceptibility in time after repeated exposure to a particular substance doesn't work with essential oils.

For common colds and flu, an inhalant made from 2 drops each of lavender, peppermint, tea tree, and eucalyptus in spring or distilled water will do the trick. A drink concocted by mixing one teaspoon of honey and one drop of essential oil mixture (1 drop of clove + 2 drops of lavender) in a cup of hot water is also a good option.

For mouth ulcers, dilute two drops of geranium, thyme, and peppermint and four drops of lemon in 2 teaspoons of brandy. Next, get one teaspoon of this mixture and add in warm water. Use the solution as mouthwash and don't swallow.

Candidiasis: Candidiasis is a disease primarily caused by the overgrowth of immune-opportunistic yeast known as candida Albicans. A recent study found that HMG CoA reductase, a key enzyme involved in the metabolism of mammals, plants, and even yeasts, is disrupted or shut down by the terrene component of essential oils, effectively deterring the yeasts from proliferating in overwhelming numbers.

Treatments for candidiasis using essential oils can be in the form of douche. And topical cream (for genitals) and suppositories. For douche, mix two tablespoons of cider vinegar, one drop of geranium, and 2 drops each of rosemary, tea tree, and lavender in 3 cups of warm, distilled water. Rinse the vagina with this solution once a day for three days. Next, add five drops of tea tree, chamomile, and lavender in 4 oz. of plain, whole-milk yogurt with live cultures. Use this as a cream to be applied to the vagina's interior.

For men, use as douche a solution made up of 1 drop essential oil mixture (5 drops each of tea tree and patchouli) added in 240mL of warm water. Next, dilute the same essential oil mixture of tea tree and patchouli in 2 tablespoons of grapeseed oil, and apply topically in the penis, specifically the foreskin portion.

. . .

It was diluting 32 drops each of lemon and eucalyptus and 48 drops of bergamot and lavender in 10 mL coconut oil to use an enema or suppository, which must be implanted in the colon and held for about 15 minutes.

For cancers:

Although many experts are still skeptical of the significance of essential oils' anticancer properties, there are still those who were open-minded to conduct clinical studies to prove the truth of such claims. The accomplishments done by science and research in this endeavor are indeed lacking and unstable, at least at this time. However, some studies have shown potential in giving light to the said matter, including those conducted in the 90s. Clinical trials have tested and found the substantial capability of terpenoids, a significant component of essential oils, in regressing tumors and treating the cancer disease.

Accepting the medical field about the nature of cancer as a disease dictated more by diet and lifestyle choices further strengthens the significance of essential oil's role in cancer treatment. Essential oils are plant oils. Therefore, a diet rich in plant foods like fruits and vegetables, the recommended diet for patients, obviously contains many essential oils and components, particularly cancer-fighting terpenoids. According to Charles Elson and Dennis Peffley, well-known contributors in basic oil research, the terpenoids' ability to shut down the metabolic enzyme HMG CoA reductase inhibits the growth and survival of cancer cells.

. . .

Another study presented the great value of essential oils in cancer treatment conducted by Dr. Anne-Marie Giraud-Robert, a French physician. The analysis takes place in 2009 at the 7th Scientific Aromatherapy Conference on Essential Oils, Cancer, Degenerative, and Autoimmune Diseases. Researchers concluded that essential oil treatments are of great value. Provided to 1,800 cancer patients, in conjunction with allopathic medicine, resulted in significantly higher survival rates. Compared to patients who have undergone allopathic treatment alone for similar cancer conditions. The observations were found valid on breast, colon, lung, and uterine cancers.

Dr. Giraud-Robert recommended that essential oil treatment be employed as backup care, considering that the standard treatment procedures for cancer, especially for terminal stages, are severe and naturally debilitating in physical, mental, and emotional aspects. However, the beautiful effects of essential oils are practical for the healing processes required after sessions of conventional cancer treatments.

For various types of cancer (the most common):

Choose from any of the following:
    Sandalwood
    Balsam Fir
    Tsuga
    Orange
    Peppermint
    Hyssop
    Frankincense
    Lavender
    Nutmeg

Melrose
Ginger
Cypress

Add seven drops of any of these oils in 2 tablespoons of carrier oil (nut oil, grapeseed oil, coconut oil). To be taken orally once a day.

For healing processes after chemotherapy:
To minimize the damage on skin due to radiation, dilute five drops of any of the following: sandalwood, peppermint, hyssop, or frankincense, in 2 tablespoons of carrier oil—massage on the affected area once or twice a day.

Inhale cypress or frankincense to stimulate the growth and rebuilding of white blood cells.

For nausea, dizziness, and vomiting, dilute 1 -3 drops of peppermint, ginger, or nutmeg in 2 – 3 tablespoons of carrier oil. Then, use either inhalant or massage oil (applied on the abdomen just above the navel and behind each ear).

Stress and Pain Relief

As previously mentioned, essential oils contain compounds that provide either energizing or relaxing effects to both mind and body upon inhalation, topical application, or ingestion.

· · ·

The limbic system, which is the part of the brain that triggers emotions and memories, is deeply affected by the works of essential oils. As a result, ordinary people and physicians alike reported a significant feeling of relaxation and improved moods during Aromatherapy. Pain and stress are also substantially reduced.

Pain and stress are the most common factors that trigger the release of endorphins, the brain chemicals, or neurotransmitters crucial to decreasing the brain's perception of pain and stress, much like the effects of codeine and morphine, but non-addictive. Endorphins are also known for their "runner's high" development, a euphoric or tremendously elated feeling like athletes experience during prolonged physical activity. With Aromatherapy, there is an increase of endorphins in the brain. Therefore, we feel less stress and pain.

In one study, magnetic resonance imaging (MRI) results showed that patients had undergone a staggering 63% reduction in claustrophobic episodes after being exposed to the vanilla aroma. Another study involving 122 patients in the ICU reported that the test subjects experienced much better after being administered lavender oil.

STIMULANTS/MOOD ENHANCERS
  Choose from any of the following:
Bergamot
Grapefruit
Lavender
Rosemary
Cardamom
Lemon

Coriander
Ginger
Geranium
Neroli
Palam rosa
Cypress

RELAXANTS/SEDATIVES

Choose from any of the following:
Nutmeg
Chamomile
Lemon
Geranium
Clary-sage
Vetiver
Marjoram
Lavender
Rose
Neroli
Sandalwood
Pettigraine

Dilute 30 -40 drops of any essential oils specified to 2 table-spoons of lotion or vegetable oil. Use as either inhalant or massage oil. You can also get the best from various properties of these essential oils, provided that must sum up the total drops summed up to 30 or 40.

Mental Health

. . .

The brain, as studies discovered, is constantly changing. More-over, it continues to alter with every experience. Therefore, it is safe to say that whatever we perceive through our senses can mold our brains. Our experiences can either improve or deteriorate our brains. That's why experts say that regularly playing mind games like puzzles and Sudoku can make the brain smarter.

Essential oils can stimulate the senses and the brain as well. These oils have even been utilized during meditation because it's easier to attain focus and deeper concentration when you're relaxed or energized with these fresh and sweet scents all around you. In addition, essential oils effectively reduce the negative repercussions of psychiatric problems such as depression, anxiety, and insomnia.

INSOMNIA

Choose from any of the following:
    Chamomile Roman
    Clary-sage
    Sandalwood
    Lemon
    Valerian
    Marjoram

Dilute 30 drops of any essential oils specified, or a combination of all (i.e., five drops each), to 2 tablespoons of nut or vegetable oil and massage to the whole body. You can also add four drops of the essential oil of your choice into your lukewarm bath.

. . .

DEPRESSION

Choose from any of the following:
  Grapefruit
  Tangerine
  Rose
  Geranium
  Dilute 30 drops of any essential oils specified, or a combination of all (i.e., five drops each), to 2 tablespoons of nut or vegetable oil and use as an inhalant.

MEMORY LOSS

Choose from any of the following:
  Rosemary
  Bergamot
  Basil
  Grapefruit
  Lavender
  Neroli

Dilute 30 drops of any essential oils specified, or a combination of all (i.e., five drops each), to 2 tablespoons of nut or vegetable oil and use as an inhalant. Store the resulting mixture in a small spray bottle which you can easily carry and spray wherever you are.

Hygiene and Sanitation

. . .

Maintaining hygiene and sanitation on the body and the surrounding is probably the cheapest and most foolproof way of preventing diseases. Fragrant doesn't always mean clean, but we can get the best of both worlds with essential oils. Even during ancient times, essential oils worked to kill harmful microbes in a naturally fragrant way. Despite the advancement in our chemical and industrial knowledge and skills. And despite the wide range of sanitizing products, we have today. There is a need to "go back to nature." It is the best and safest choice that we can ever have.

The aforementioned is especially sure amidst the growing health concern about the correlation of degenerative diseases such as cancers, Alzheimer's, and diabetes. We get exposed to chemicals every day and everywhere, even in the haven we call home.

Essential oils are natural antiseptics and disinfectants. They are non-toxic and very safe, at least if we smell them since the initial preparations and before topical application and ingestion of the said oils.

HAND HYGIENE

Choose from any of the following:
Tea Tree
Peppermint
Lemon
Geranium

The best way to start good hygiene and maintain sanitized conditions is by washing hands at least every 30 minutes. Diluting 30 drops of any listed essential oils (or a combination of each) in 10mL distilled water or 5mL aloe vera gel would be a powerful hand sanitizer. It will surely kill the germs while still care for the skin, keeping it always moisturized.

MOUTH HYGIENE (TEETH AND GUMS)

32

Choose from any of the following:

Peppermint
   Lemon
   Orange
   Myrrh

For Mouthwash:

Dilute two drops of any of the essential oils listed above in 1 tablespoon of vodka.

Store the solution in a glass bottle.

Get five drops of this mixture and dilute it with a glass of water.

Use as a mouthwash.

For tooth powder: Gather the following ingredients:

. . .

1 tbsp. Dry orange or banana peel, ground
   2 tsp. Dry sage, ground
   2 tsp. Soda Bicarbonate or Arrowroot flour
   1 tsp. Salt

Combine the ingredients. Add five drops of lemon and one drop of peppermint to the mixture. Mix well. Place on toothbrush and rub on the teeth. Don't swallow.

BODY HYGIENE

Choose from any of the following:
   Clary-sage
   Thyme
   Peppermint
   Eucalyptus
   Sage

Dilute five drops of eucalyptus and peppermint, 15 drops of sage, and ten drops of thyme in 2 tablespoons of base oil. Store the solution in a glass bottle. Apply on the whole body after taking a bath.

Food and Cooking

The natural fragrance and stimulating properties of essential oils would be a complete waste if we won't grasp them. Although such properties are not tangible, we can somehow own them by experiencing such wonders are the food we enjoy. Various recipes' zesty flavor can only be made possible by plant ingredients like herbs and spices. Such characteristics are given life by the essential oils naturally contained in them.

When adding essential oils to recipes, the rule of thumb is to add only toward the end of the final baking. Then, simmering, or boiling process to take advantage of their aroma and flavor since these oils are highly volatile, and they'll be gone in a whiff if exposed in extreme temperatures. The recommended amount for essential oils is 2 – 3 drops.

However, there is great concern about the safety of ingesting concentrated amounts of essential oils, which experts recommend time and again as something to be avoided at all costs. Essential oils, as the Food and Drug Administration (FDA) declared, must be used for our food as additives or flavoring only.

LIST OF FDA-APPROVED ESSENTIAL OILS FOR FOOD ADDITIVES

Bergamot
    Grapefruit
    Lavender
    Rosemary
    Basil
    Lemon
    Chamomile (Roman and German)
    Ginger
    Geranium
    Neroli

Galbanum
Jasmine
Nutmeg
Sage
Spearmint
Tarragon
Lemongrass
Patchouli
Oregano
Cinnamon
Lime
Tangerine
Thyme
Peppermint
Clove
Dill
Hyssop
Orange
Valerian
Coriander
Ylang Ylang
Petitgrain
Rose
Sandalwood
Pine
Eucalyptus

Home Use

The only place where we could fully enjoy and be comfortable is our home. More than to be habitable for ourselves and entertaining and homely for our guests, we all like our homes to be clean, fragrant, and beautifully decorated. Not just appearance, but the aroma, can say a lot about the type of people living in a house. Hence, aside from the homey feels of baked bread or brewed coffee that we let our guests (and prospective house buyers) experience, why not spray a mist of lemon or rose or clary-sage to make people, guests, and house residents alike feel relaxed and comfortable.

Using essential oils is a natural, practical, and safe way of making your home more than just a livable shack. Aside from the wide range of delightful aromas you can choose from and experiment on, we all have learned that essential oils contain natural and non-toxic antiseptic, anti-depressive, analgesic, and detoxifying properties. They are also highly versatile; you can store them anywhere in the kitchen, terrace, garden, garage, bathroom, and bedrooms.

For Air Fresheners:

Choose any essential oil you want.
Add eight drops of essential oil to 2½ cups of distilled/spring water.
Store the solution in a spray bottle.
Spray in the air, curtains, ceiling, and empty spaces.
Avoid spraying on spots and corners where staining can occur, say, on velvet materials and wood furniture.
Do this specially to remove the smells of cooking.

For Disinfectants: Most of the essential oils available commercially possess potent antiseptic and bactericide properties. But the classic favorites for home disinfection are eucalyptus, peppermint, lemon, thyme, lavender, pine, clove, and grapefruit.

Just add 2 – 5 drops on a wet cloth and use it to wipe the parts of the house where harmful microbes usually hang out. These include the kitchen sink, the toilet seat, kitchen and bathroom floors, and the dining table. Next, add three drops of essential oil to a basin of warm water (about 60 - 70°C), and sterilize your kitchenware, especially the eating utensils, for 10 – 15 minutes.

For Pest Repellents:

To deter creepy crawlies, rodents, and other uninvited guests from entering your humble abode, be sure that you have any of the following: lavender, rosemary, thyme, lemongrass, citronella, basil, cinnamon, and peppermint. Wet a cotton ball or a cloth with ten drops of any essential oil of your choice (in concentrated amounts) and wipe the places where these pests thrive or probably enter. You can also apply some on paper strips and put these strips on windowsills, kitchen doors, and cupboard linings.

Weight Loss

Recent studies are trying to explore the significance of Aromatherapy in weight loss – an idea that logically followed the research that found essential oils, like those extracted from lemon and grapefruit, to aid in the faster metabolism of fats. In contrast, more investigations and clinical experiments work to shed more light on this subject. And finally, make such a concept unchallenged. Some studies showed potential, proving that the connection between essential oil properties and weight maintenance is not entirely impossible.

5

CONCOCTING YOUR ESSENTIAL OIL MIX FOR DIFFERENT PURPOSES

Different types and brands of essential oils are commercially available. You can find them anywhere, even in small grocery stores. Most of the product's indispensable in our everyday daily life also contain essential oils. Despite this convenience, many still are die-hard DIY lovers, and well, you can never really go wrong if you start from scratch. Most importantly, you can be in complete control of experimenting and getting the best results if you prepare the raw materials and create the masterpiece independently.

When handling essential oils, you can concoct your mixture or even extract the essential oil itself by following some basic guides designed and practiced by connoisseurs. Essential oils can be expensive, but extraction and concoction activities at home can be highly pocket friendly.

Extraction

. . .

Extraction of essential oils can help in various ways that will require only the basic knowledge you learned in your elementary science class. Most of the techniques we have today, even sophisticated ones, are just improved from the crude methods our ancestors initially perform.

One such method is the enfleurage, which probably isn't practiced anywhere anymore except in France. In this method, flower blossoms are arranged on sheets of warm animal fat or vegetable oil to incorporate their fragrance and essence into the fat.

Another is by expression, which is the most straightforward way of obtaining essential oils. In this method, the plant parts containing the desired essential oil, including the gum resins, skins, flesh, seeds, leaves, and flowers, are pressed manually or mechanically with such force until the essential oils or the plant fluids contain the vital oils seep out. This procedure can't be done as a solo method but must be performed instead as an initial method before distillation, another extraction method.

The most employed and popular method of essential oil extraction today is probably distillation. This procedure considers that crucial oils can mix and form one phase with other oils and fats and readily dissolve in alcohol but never in water. This method requires a distillation set-up commonly referred to as stills.

There are ingredients or stills for essential oil extraction purchased from stores and set up at home. This equipment can be a bit high-priced, but if you plan to make essential oils as your lifetime hobby or probably a business venture, then consider purchasing them as a long-term investment. On the other hand, if you're a start-from-scratch fan, you can avail every part of the equipment and build the still bit by bit. Finally, a standard still is designed and formed, as seen in the figure below. Though a rough illustration of a still, you get the picture.

The critical components of a still include a heat source. Probably a large stove or furnace to provide fire which will boil the water. A retort or holding tank with a built-in (or accessorized) grate can place the plant material. A condenser will collect the steam and condense it through piping immersed in cold water, and a separator, also known as the essence, will separate the essential oil from the water vapor.

However, before carrying out the distillation process, you must know the main categories of essential oils based on their volatility. These categories are the top, middle and base notes. The top notes that essential oils are the quickest to volatilize, usually lasting for 3 to 24 hours. The middle notes are moderately volatile, with complete evaporation lasting to a maximum of 3 days. Essential oils of this type can affect bodily functions, particularly metabolism. The base note's last classification includes essential oils that are slower to volatilize, usually lasting to almost a week before entirely evaporating. These oils are generally those with highly soothing properties, and therefore the most relaxing.

Concoction

When making your essential oil recipe mix, always remember that these oils can be highly irritating and sensitizing to the skin in concentrated amounts. That's why it is better to dilute these oils in another fluid medium before use. The most common diluents are distilled water and base oils. Base oils or what others call carrier oils can be animal fats or plant oils. Plant-based oils can be seed oils, nuts oils, and vegetable oils. The user can purchase some of them, but you can also extract them on your own. Examples are olive oil, avocado oil, apricot kernel oil, coconut oil, sesame oil, corn oil, jojoba oil, grape seed oil, and wheat germ oil.

If you purchase essential oils for a specific use, knowing their quality will prepare you financially because the best quality has the highest price. When choosing essential oils, you must look for purity, grade, and integrity.

Purity

Purity is a quality that is too hard to find these days since the economic talks of money and revenues always get in the way of providing the public with high-quality yet safe products. However, not everything labeled as "100% pure" is true. And with the continuous advancement in clinical technologies and laboratory techniques, synthetic substances and chemicals coming even in something delicate as food are more than a possibility – it's a reality that's happening every day. Even burger patties now can be made straight from the lab.

The danger of commercially available essential oils is dependent mainly on purity. Adulterated brands cut or worse. Entirely replaced by cheaper laboratory-made substitutes are expectedly not as potent as the original and probably hazardous or toxic to health. So, such inexpensive oils like orange or peppermint are altered, and of course, it's entirely the opposite with expensive ones like rose and jasmine.

The purity of an essential oil can't be easy to determine by just visual inspection and even by touch. For example, while vegetable oil-diluted oils are easy to find, those dissolved in alcohol are different since alcohols are clear and non-oily solvents.

Grades

Scents physically determine the grades of essential oils. Those with higher rates, which are more expensive, are more concentrated and therefore more intense, fragrance-wise. A higher concentration is obtained. by repeating the extraction process, such as the re-distillation procedure.

Integrity

A brand made of pure essential oil, but the next question is the integrity, which pertains to the oil's purity of origin, i.e., the botanical source from where it comes. An essential oil obtained from a single plant species that thrive in a specific region and presents itself commercially as a genuine true to its origin, it possesses high-class integrity. Due to cost constraints, there are cheaper essential oils that, albeit in unadulterated form, are combined with other pure essential oils and manipulated to pose as an alternative to an expensive type of essential oil. For instance, lemongrass essential oils are usually used in the lab to mimic the costly lemon balm or melissa oil. While you may be relieved about the purity of such essential oils, low integrity will not give your desired and expected results.

6

MORE TIPS TO REMEMBER ABOUT ESSENTIAL OILS AND THEIR USES

Always remember the following details when dealing with essential oils:

1. While distilled water is a suitable diluent if you're aiming for an essential oil spray, the best option to get the desired consistency and mixing of your final product is by using vegetable oil as a diluent instead. Therefore, always keep a jar or bottle of veggie oil handy.

2. Essential oils are concentrated in pure form, and while they are botanically sourced and non-toxic, erroneous applications and preparations can result in events detrimental to both life and health. Hence, a recommendation is to consult an essential oil expert with a physician's background and authority before trying any of these oils out. This precaution is particularly crucial for children, pregnant or lactating women, and people with special conditions like epilepsy, schizophrenia, and high blood pressure.

. . .

3. To lengthen the shelf life of essential oils, store them in dark glass bottles with tight lids. Please keep them in a cold, dry place, away from light, because they can be sensitive to it since these oils are organic. Therefore, we can be sure that their most effective state can last up to 2 years only. However, some essential oils, like wine, become more fragrant and potent as they age. An example of such oil is eucalyptus.

4. Essential oils applied topically can increase the susceptibility of the skin to UV exposure. Don't forget to apply sunblock before basking in the sunlight.

5. Practice extreme care when using essential oils. The thin area under the eyes is off-limits. Don't put oils inside the ears. Wash your hands with crucial oil first before eating food or cleaning your contacts.

6. To test for allergies, apply a small amount on the forearm and check if any marks, rash, or itchiness occurs within 24 hours.

7. There might be essential oils that are safe to ingest, but it wouldn't hurt to partner with honey or soy milk to neutralize any harsh effects of essential oils when taken internally.

8. Mix in drops of essential oils to a bath gel base or plant base oils before adding to a water bath.

9. Avoid the following plant oils at all costs: wormwood, rue, bitter almond, horseradish, sassafras, mustard, pennyroyal tea,

mugwort, wintergreen, boldo leaf, thuja, wormseed, tansy, yellow camphor, calamus, southernwood, and savin.

AFTERWORD

I hope this book was able to help you to understand and be excited about essential oils and their healthy wonders. Essential oils have been around us since ancient times, not only perfuming the air we breathe but also providing a wide range of uses that benefit our homes, family, environment, and life.

It's also one of the most enjoyable hobbies. Unfortunately, we don't get much chance to unleash the scientist and magician in us with all the daily business and busyness. However, such an opportunity is more than possible when concocting different recipes for essential oils that will suit our needs.

The next step is to make a list of essential oils with the ones you want to experiment with, ask an expert first before the concoction proper. As much as essential oils are well-regarded for their therapeutic potential, they can significantly give devastating effects if misused and handled carelessly. We must never forget that essential oils must come from botanical materials that are otherwise safe and non-toxic. Still, these oils sometimes are naturally packed with complex chemical components and soothing properties.

Aromatherapy is not used or widely trusted (particularly by physicians) in the mainstream medical field. Although they firmly believe in chemically synthesized drugs and sophisticated medical procedures and equipment. No one can reject that its natural outlook towards disease prevention and treatment makes it one of the safest, effective, and probably cheapest ways of maintaining optimum health. A reason why essential oils have been present in the past and used by the experts today is history attesting that such oils' utilization was not just by whim because it has transcended across ages and geographical barriers.

Aromatherapy, however, is just one side of the multi-faceted approach to achieving health and longevity. It may be effective, and right now, a good bud in the medical field. However, it's still just a part of a bigger picture occupied by a balanced diet, healthy habits, lifestyle, regular meditation, and happiness.
The End.

Did you like this book? Then you'll LOVE Perfect Evernote: The Best Tips You Have to know

Keeping track of ideas, notes, grocery lists, interesting websites, or whatever can be a never ending rask.
You can try using a word processor or even a spreadsheet.
Sure these programs will do the trick when you first start off but when you start to expand and start gathering tons of information the task can be overwhelming.
This is why I am telling you about this great program Evernote.
Evernote is a free application that handles all of your notes and information in a single location with unlimited storage and incredible search features.
In this book we will explore the basics of Evernote and what it does and what you can do with it.
It is our goal that once you complete this book that you will have

a full understanding of what Evernote is and what it can do for you and your life.

Evernote is an amazing app which is the best program to organize your entire life and can also help in completing any task and accomplishing your goals.

Evernote is the best thing there is to help you crush it in your goals.

This Evernote guide will teach you the basics you have to know in order to make the most of this great program

Perfect Evernote: The Best Tips You Have to know

https://books2read.com/u/bo8M0Z

Perfect Evernote: The Best Tips You Have to know

https://books2read.com/u/bo8M0Z

———

SO, WHAT IS EVERNOTE?

Evernote is, in my opinion, the ultimate note-taking and collaboration application that you can use. Evernote allows you, the end-user, to take notes, collaborate with others, share ideas, find information, and much, much more with just a few clicks of the mouse or swipes of your finger.

Evernote can be found on the following website.

http://www.evernote.com. The application is free, and one account can be accessed from an unlimited number of locations such as PC, Mac, Android, iPhone, Web, and more. Evernote has a premium account that is $4.99 a month or $49.99 a year at the time of this writing. With the premium version, you will have access to more advanced features, but these features are not needed for everyday users.

LET'S GET STARTED

Okay, let's jump right in with both feet. The first thing that you will want to do is visit the Evernote website by visiting http://www.evernote.com

From there, you will see a button that says "Download". Click on this link to get the software.

CREATING AN ACCOUNT

Once you download the software and install it, I downloaded my copy for the Android system; you will be required to create an account.

CHOOSE YOUR ACCOUNT TYPE

The first step is to choose your account type. At the time of this writing, there are three account types Free, Premium, and Business. For this book, we will be focusing on the free account of Evernote.

. . .

In the Premium account, you will get the ability to have one gig of file storage each month. This means that each month you will receive one gig of storage that accumulates.

So if you have one gig of files in January, you automatically get another one gig of storage in February, which will total two gigs of notes. In addition, you will get additional features such as the ability to password protect files and many other support and premium features.

The business account option is similar, but it gives you the option of having four gigs of storage space compared to the one gig in the personal account and the option to collaborate with others.

Before choosing to pay for any account access, it is strongly suggested that you first start with the free account, get your feet wet in the Evernote universe, and upgrade once you know what it can do and what it will do for you.

USERNAME AND PASSWORD

Creating an account is very simple. The only information that is required is a username and a password.

The username will be your e-mail address. When creating your account, make sure you use a legitimate e-mail address. It can be an e-mail address that you don't use, or you can set up an e-mail account specifically for Evernote, but you will need to have a real e-mail address that functions to create your account.

The password you choose should be strongly phrased.

The password should be unique and not something you use for other accounts. You will want to use letters, numbers, uppercase, lowercase, and don't have anything in sequential order. Take note of your passwords, and don't allow others to access them.

If someone has your username and password, they will have access to your account and can damage or use your personal information against you.

Once you have created an account, it will be time to log in and start using all the great features. In the next chapter, we will go through all of the basic features you get with Evernote and show you how to create notebooks, notes, and much more. Then in chapter three, we will explore some add-ons and other more advanced features that will be available in the premium and business versions. We will give you some additional information and ideas for using evermore in the final chapter.

End of Sneak Peek.

Perfect Evernote: The Best Tips You Have to know

https://books2read.com/u/bo8M0Z